Lose Your Belly Diet:

Get That Flat Tummy!

Table of Contents

that may befall them after undertaking information described herein.

Additionally, the information in the following pages is intended only for informational purposes and should thus be thought of as universal. As befitting its nature, it is presented without assurance regarding its prolonged validity or interim quality. Trademarks that are mentioned are done without written consent and can in no way be considered an endorsement from the trademark holder.

Introduction

Congratulations on getting this book and thank you for doing so.

The following chapters will discuss all the little things you can do to make sure that you get rid of that annoying belly fat and learn how to live your best life with the healthiest eating choices.

Thanks again for choosing this book. Every effort was made to ensure it is full of as much useful information as possible, please enjoy!

Chapter 1: What Causes Belly Fat to Build Up?

There are many reasons that belly fat may build up. Most of these have to do with the way you live your life, the things you eat and how you take care of your gut. For most people, a buildup of belly fat isn't just from one thing but is, instead, from a combination of several things they probably did wrong throughout their lives.

Belly fat is not only a huge inconvenience and something most people are embarrassed about, but it is something that is unhealthy. Having a lot of belly fat can put you at risk for some of the worst diseases, can lead to stroke and can even cause you to die, long before it is your time to die. There are many implications of having a lot of belly fat, but the *Lose Your Belly Diet* is one that is aimed at making you more comfortable in your own skin and getting rid of the fat that separates you from a happy life.

Sugar
One of the biggest causes of people carrying around excess weight, especially around their belly, is too much sugar in their diet. Sugar is a nutrient and something that you might always need, especially if you are going to eat fruit and stay healthy. But, it is also something that can be very detrimental to your health. Sugar can contribute to heart disease and diabetes, along with causing a slew of other problems. Those who consume too much sugar aren't usually even the people with a "sweet tooth," who eat cake for breakfast, but are more commonly people who eat a lot of processed foods. Sugar is

hidden in a lot of different foods and this can be a problem because you're eating a ton of it. You just don't realize there is a problem with what you're eating, so you just continue to eat it.

Lack of Sleep

If you think missing a few hours of sleep each night isn't going to do much damage to you, other than cause you to throw back an extra coffee in the morning, you're critically wrong. A lack of sleep can contribute to things like physical exhaustion but it can also cause you to carry extra weight around. When you do not sleep enough, you will have a buildup of cortisol, which can cause you to gain weight or not be able to lose weight. Try going to bed one hour earlier every night to get an added 7 hours of sleep per week – that's almost like getting an extra night of sleep!

Not Moving

Most people realize that not exercising can contribute to belly fat and a buildup of weight, but what if you put your 30 minutes in at the gym every day and you're still not seeing results? The problem comes from being inactive. If you have a desk job or a job that does not require you to move around a lot, or if you simply just don't move around other than that 30 minutes in the gym, it is not doing any good. Consider taking a quick five minute walk around the office, every hour or two, to help get your heart pumping and you'll begin to see some of the belly fat slide right off.

Alcohol

Along with other foods that have secret sugars, alcohol is one of the biggest offenders. Many people realize that their nightly drink routine could be hurting their waistline, but what they don't realize is that there is something they can do about it. By cutting out just one drink per day, you can see a weight loss of up to 14 pounds per year. If you are unable to cut that out or if you only drink one drink per day, consider switching it for something that doesn't have quite as much sugar in it.

Stress

When you don't get enough sleep, your body releases too much cortisol, which is in response to the stress your body is under when you are exhausted. This can happen with any type of stress, whether it is from a lack of sleep, family problems or even just daily life. When you work to reduce the stress in your life, you will be able to release less cortisol. You'll see a huge change in the way your body works, and you'll even notice that you are not holding onto as much belly fat. Because of the way cortisol works, the hormones cause the fat to build up in the middle of your body – right in your belly.

Not Enough Protein

It is important to have a diet rich in protein that comes from lean sources. If you are not getting enough protein, chances are that you are hungry most of the day and you eat more to compensate for it. While you need other nutrients in your life to be able to survive, protein is very important. It will help you to stay full, can help contribute to stronger muscles and will allow you to get the best nutrition possible. Those that switch from a diet that is high in carbs or high in fat, to a diet that is lower in each of those things and higher in protein, will see bigger results when they step on the scale. It is important to note that you cannot live on protein alone and that you should consider adding some fats and carbohydrates to your diet, but do so in a way that is healthy for your body.

Trans Fat
Fat is absolutely not the worst thing in the world for you, but trans fat actually can be. Trans fat is a type of manufactured fat. It is created when hydrogen is added to fat, to help keep the fat stable longer. This is something done in packaged foods and prepared meals that causes them to be high in trans fat and allows them to stay shelf-stable for a longer time. If you cut down on processed foods when you are trying to lose belly fat, you will see a huge difference in your body in a short amount of time.

Your Family
If you have a large belly, you may be able to thank your dear old mom or dad for that. Genetics do play a large role in the way people carry weight, how obese they are and how they lose weight. If someone's parents are overweight, he or she is more likely to be overweight, not only because he or she is likely eating food that is bad for them, but also because he or she has genetics that are predisposed to being overweight or obese. The good news is that healthy eating can, for the most part, beat genetics.

Fruit Juices
Your morning routine of orange juice before heading into work could also be contributing to the belly fat you are carrying around. Fruit juices are one of the foods that you may not expect to be, but are actually loaded with sugar. The secret sugar in fruit juice can cause you to hold onto your weight, make you not lose any weight and

contribute to a slew of health problems. If you are drinking fruit juice, at any point throughout the day, consider swapping it for something like water or tea that is lower in calories with no sugar or added chemical/preservatives.

Low Fiber

Fiber is important to keep your body functioning. If your diet is low in fiber, you may not be losing as much weight as you would like it to be. Try adding some different sources of fiber to your diet, to make sure that you get the most fiber possible. This can also help you in other areas of your health as well. For fibrous meals, consider trying things like whole grain bread, whole wheat pasta and oats. These are minor changes that can allow you to see big differences, when compared to the white versions of these foods.

Hormonal Changes

If you are going through menopause or having any other hormonal changes, it could be what your belly fat problems are all about. While there is nothing that you can do to stop menopause, there are a few things you can do to battle the belly fat that comes along with it. Be sure you are eating healthy and continuing to exercise throughout menopause, so you will be better able to manage the belly fat that comes along with it.

Gut Problems

Inside of you, there are millions of bacteria and thousands of different types of bacteria. If you have been eating an unhealthy diet for any length of time, the chances are high that you could have more unhealthy bacteria in your gut than the healthy kind. Not only will bad bacteria make you feel run down, bloated and just uncomfortable, but it can also contribute to belly fat. If you want to get good bacteria back into your gut, consider eating fermented food, like yogurt and other things that contain bacteria in them. The good bacteria will eventually overpower the bad and you will be able to have a healthier gut, contributing to a healthier life and a smaller belly.

Chapter 2: Gut Damage? What to Do?

Many people have a damaged gut and don't even know it. This can come from a buildup of bad bacteria in the gut and can make it difficult for you to be able to lose any weight or get rid of any of the fat you are carrying. Because of the way that gut damage works, it can cause you to feel tired all the time and can contribute to other problems like both physical and mental diseases. A bad gut or one that is high in bad bacteria can cause major health problems.

Your bathroom habits are one of the biggest indicators of whether you have a healthy gut. If you defecate on a regular basis and it is similar in consistency each time you go, chances are that you have a healthy gut. If your bathroom habits are more varied, such that you have to go more often one day and not at all the next, or if the consistency varies from day to day, your gut is probably in distress and needs some good bacteria to help it get better, so you can get back to "normal."

It is common for people who have a lot of belly fat to also have gut damage. This is because both belly fat and gut damage are results of a very unhealthy diet. While they are not always completely related, they might go hand in hand with each other because of the problems they cause and because of the things they are a result of. It is important to note that the belly fat you see doesn't always mean you have a gut problem, but the chances are high that your gut could be damaged from eating many years' worth of bad food.

Another indicator that can be a sign of a bad gut, is the way your moods vary. If you have mood swings, if you get very happy or sad on a regular basis, or if you have trouble controlling your mood, your gut may be in bad shape. It may seem strange to think of your gut having a problem and your mood showing it, but it is certainly something the gut can impact. If your body is not functioning at its optimum level, then your mind won't be functioning the way it is supposed to either.

As you figure out if you have a bad gut or not, you will also be able to figure out how you can fix it. Having bad bacteria in your gut, isn't the end of the world. The good news is that it is relatively simple to fix a bad gut or the bad bacteria in your gut, with just a few dietary changes. The point of each of these is to get good bacteria back into your gut and try to allow it to begin functioning in the way it is supposed to. All you need to do is follow the four R's of healing a bad gut, and you will be well on your way to better gut health, a happier life and a smaller belly.

Remove
The first thing you should do, when you are going to try to fix your gut health, is remove the foods and toxins that are hurting your gut. This is something that can be difficult, especially for people who are accustomed to eating a regular, modern diet, but as you learn more about the different things you can do, it will help your gut health to improve.

You should first make sure you remove the things that are not food items and are causing toxic buildups in your gut. These are things like medications that have not been prescribed by your doctor. Ibuprofen, acetaminophen and even antacids can all contribute to bad bacteria in your gut. After about a week of not consuming any of these things, you will notice that your gut is already much better and is beginning to heal. But, this is not the only thing that you should remove out of your diet.

You need to try your hardest to remove all processed foods from your diet. While it is not necessarily harmful to have a processed food occasionally, most people are consuming large amounts of processed foods on a daily basis. This is something the body was not intended to be able to handle and something that has made many people very sick. For the sake of simplicity, processed food is anything that has more than five ingredients in it or has ingredients that you are unable to pronounce.

It is a good idea to remove all processed foods from your diet because they can be the contributing factor that is causing bad bacteria in the gut. But, you will also need to do things that will allow you to repair your gut. When you have stopped eating processed foods and toxins that can make you feel bad, you will immediately start to feel better. It usually starts within the first few days and it will only get better, as you go through the process of changing your diet to one that is good for your gut.

Repair

After you have cut the processed food out of your diet, you need to work on repairing your gut, so you will be able to complete the program. This can take anywhere from two to four weeks and will depend on the way you feel. You need to get in tune with your body and learn the signals it is giving you. Depending on the progress of the repair, you may need to stay in this stage for a little longer than you were expecting.

Once you have taken the processed foods out of your diet, allow your body to rest by feeding it only natural and completely unprocessed foods. Give it fruits, vegetables and whole grains. Consider making your own things, like bread and Greek yogurt, which are both very easy to make, and will allow you to feel better as soon as you start to eat them. Eating a comforting diet during this time will give the gut a chance to start to heal and continue losing weight because of the way the foods are created and what they are able give you.

When you are at this stage, you will also want to eat foods that are going to contribute to repair. Probiotics and prebiotics are both beneficial to your gut health. These are found in things like Greek yogurt and other cultured food; just make sure that you are not eating the over processed versions of each. It is easy to make your own Greek yogurt and kefir, so now would be the time to try it. You should also be eating things like turmeric and mint on your food, to help your stomach feel better and give your gut the chance to heal as much as possible.

Once you have fully repaired your gut, you will want to continue with the last two R's. You will know your gut has been repaired when your bathroom habits become more regular, when you stop feeling so bloated and when you feel like you can eat food without getting sick or without any complications, like running to the bathroom each time you eat. It is a good idea to take as long as possible in the repair stage, if you are unsure of whether or not your gut have been fully repaired.

Restore

When you are sure that your gut is repaired and you do not have any lingering problems from your previous poor diet, you can begin to restore it. You should only do this after you are sure that your gut has repaired itself, as this will allow you the chance to make sure you are getting the most from the process. One thing to note is that the restore stage is where people usually go wrong, because of the delicate balance you need to restore to your gut and the way it can cause you to start eating unhealthily again.

It is a good idea to try doing this first with probiotic yogurt. Since you should have already made your own Greek yogurt in the previous step, you should ramp up the amount you are eating. The probiotics in the yogurt are the good bacteria, which will allow you to build up more bacteria in your gut, in order to to combat the bad bacteria in the future. When you consume the Greek yogurt, it will allow you the chance to make sure you are getting the best bacteria possible.

If you do not like yogurt, you do not have the time to make your own or you are unable to eat it for whatever reason, you can purchase probiotic supplements. These often come in pill form or even chewable form. They are a great addition to your supplements and will allow you the chance to make sure you are getting the most out of your diet and the best possible bacteria in your gut. You can also consume these to help keep you healthier during "flu seasons" or times when people get sick very often.

This step is also the step in which you will be able to add other things back into your diet, like meat and other sources of protein. While they are not as good as probiotics at bringing good bacteria in, they have their own place in being able to add bacteria back to your gut. They are a great way for you to be able to get the bacteria you need and they will be your best source of protein. Lean meat is the best for making sure you can lose belly fat. Organic and natural meats will also help you to be as healthy as possible.

Replace
There are some things you will need to replace after you have healed your gut. These are things like the acid in your stomach and other types of flora that may be present in your gut. You need to make sure you are replacing them after you have healed your gut because they could be deleted both from your restoration and from your previous bad eating habits. To replace them, you will need to eat foods that are nutrient rich.

Start out by adding more vegetables to your diet. Try vegetables that are fermented too because they will help your gut replace some of the things it may be missing. However, be careful with fermented vegetables. Do not eat too many of them at one time because they can occasionally have bad bacteria in them and can begin to harm you again, like you were harmed when you had bad eating habits. Finding the delicate balance is something you will need to do, in order to be able to maintain the best gut health possible.

This is also the stage when you will begin to eat a lot of fruit again. The fruit can have exactly what you need to make sure you are going to get all of the healthy things in your gut, because of the unique way it is able to help contribute to nutrients. When you eat fruit, you should make sure you are consuming the good kind. Don't eat fruit that has been processed. If you cannot get to a fresh source of fruit, frozen fruits are acceptable but canned fruits are not.

As you go through each of these things, you may find that your gut has not started to replace everything you need. You may need to push it along with digestive enzyme supplements and even things like papaya extract, which can both help to heal your gut. They will help to replace the things you have lost and allow you the chance to make sure you are getting the best possible experience out of the healing process. You need to make sure you are able to have good digestive health, if you want to maintain the healthy gut you just worked so hard to get.

Chapter 3: What Food to Eat in this Diet Plan?

Now that you have learned the things you *shouldn't* be eating (processed foods), we will need to go over each of the things you *should* be eating to make the fat burning diet plan better able to work with your body and get rid of the belly fat you have built up throughout the time you were eating bad food and living an unhealthy lifestyle.

There is no exact plan telling you what food you can and cannot eat. There are certain foods that should be avoided and certain foods you should eat more of, but this is not a fad diet that tells you "only eat cottage cheese for three weeks" or "never even smell a carb again." The difference between this plan and those is that this is meant to change your lifestyle, your mindset and your attitude toward food – for the long term.

Protein

The most important part of the *Lose Your Belly Diet* is that you are going to eat a lot of protein. That is why it is one of the first things you will need to put back into your diet, when you have healed your gut, and why it will continue to be able to help you lose fat. Protein is exactly what your body needs to be able to get the fuel it needs to continue going. Unlike carbohydrates or other nutrients, protein is converted directly to fuel.

You should make sure you are eating lean protein as much as possible because that is what is going to help you lose the most belly fat. Do not gorge yourself on high-fat ground beef or other fatty foods. You should try to eat chicken, turkey, lean cuts of steak, salmon and other fish. The best food to eat, to get the protein you need, is poultry (which includes eggs) because it does not have the fat content that red meat does, but it *does* have a protein that is comparable. When you are eating a lot of poultry, you get a lot of lean protein, without all the negatives that come with red meat.

No matter what type of lean protein you are going to choose to eat, you should make sure it is either natural, organic or both. This will guarantee that nothing has been added to it and it is not very processed. Stay away from lean protein that has been fried, cooked in trans fat or has anything added to it because it will hurt your belly fat situation, instead of being able to help make you lose it like you want to.

Vegetables
Eating your vegetables is one of the best ways you can make sure you are going to heal your gut and get rid of your belly fat. Vegetables are both packed with nutrients and very filling. The vegetables you consume should be as fresh as possible and should help you get rid of your belly fat. If you eat canned vegetables, you are going to be eating the preservatives that contributed to your belly fat and the bad gut problems you had, before you healed it. Make sure you are eating vegetables that are as fresh as possible.

There are some vegetables that may not be the best choice for you when you are trying to lose belly fat. While all vegetables may have a trace amount of carbohydrates in them, you should steer clear of the ones that have a lot of carbs. Limit your intake of potatoes and corn because of the carb content. This can cause problems for your gut and could make you blow the *Lose Your Belly Diet* you have worked so hard. It is a good idea to focus instead on leafy green vegetables.

Tomatoes, peppers, eggplant and other nightshade plants may also pose a problem when you are doing the *Lose Your Belly Diet*. While these don't necessarily have a lot of carbs in them, they can be detrimental because of the family they come from. They are often very hard on the stomach and can cause you to have problems. If you have just healed your gut, you may want to wait for a little while before you try to eat these vegetables. Otherwise, you may bring harm to the place you just tried to heal through the various methods included with the four R's.

Fruits

Throughout the time you are doing the *Lose Your Belly Diet*, the fruit you eat is going to help you stay on track. Fruit is nature's dessert, but it also has other health benefits. No matter your reason for eating fruit, you can make sure you are having the best *Lose Your Belly Diet* experience by adding fruit to your diet and replacing some of the other things you eat with fruit, so you are able to get the most out of the process and lose the most belly fat possible.

If you are craving something sweet, your first instinct should be to reach for fruit. Once you have cut out the processed food and refined sugar, fruit will begin to taste very sweet. You can try different varieties and even add exotic fruit to your diet. This is something that will allow you the chance to make sure you are making good decisions. Fruit will help to keep you from going back to your old eating habits and ruining the diet you worked so hard on.

Even if you are eating some non-plant based fiber, the fruit will probably be your biggest source of fiber. Most fruit is very fibrous and will allow you to get the fiber you need to be able to survive. Things like berries, bananas and apples come with a lot of fiber. They will help you feel better. They will contribute to the loss of belly fat and provide you with healthy fiber that you absolutely need.

Fat
While trans fat is not good for you, there are other types of fat that can help you live a happy and healthy life while you are doing the *Lose Your Belly Diet.* The fat you consume should be combined with protein and should contribute to helping you feel fuller for longer periods of time. There are some natural, non-animal sources of fat that will also help you feel better and get the best nutrition possible. It is a good idea to try these, to make sure you are getting the most out of the *Lose Your Belly Diet,* so you will feel better and lose weight.

The most common fat you are going to eat, when you are doing the *Lose Your Belly Diet,* will come from protein sources. While chicken and other types of poultry do not have a lot of fat in them, they will still provide some of it. Lean red meat, pork and some fish have more fat in them, will help you to feel better and keep you fuller longer with the combination of the protein included in each of these sources.

Plant sources of fat include things like avocados. They have a lot of fat in them but it's the good fat. The fat you eat should be natural, should be easy to digest and should *never* be processed, like trans fat.

Fiber

Fiber works in combination with protein to help keep you full. Fiber is great, especially in the morning when you combine it with protein, because it will keep you full throughout the day. While you don't necessarily want to skip meals, eating a breakfast that has protein and fiber in it will allow you to skip the morning snack you may be used to.

The majority of your fiber is going to come from fruit. While fruit is filled with sugar and carbs, it is also filled with fiber. The fiber can help cancel out the negative effects of the sugar and the carbs, because of the way it works with the body. It will allow you the chance to make sure you are getting the most protein possible. When you consume the protein and fiber together, you will be able to do something like a sausage, avocado and grapefruit breakfast. This will keep you fuller for much longer than just throwing back an egg and croissant sandwich from your local fast food restaurant.

You can also get fiber from sources like whole grain bread, whole grain pasta and other whole grain carbs. While the carbs you consume in these forms aren't as harmless as they are in fruit, the fiber will help to make them easier for you to digest. If you are going to consume carbs in the form of bread, you need to make sure you are doing it with a lot of fiber, only consuming sources that are high in fiber.

Low Carbohydrates

It can be detrimental to your body to completely cut out carbohydrates from your diet. You will still want to eat them in things like fruit and even fibrous foods like whole wheat bread. Cutting carbs completely out will eliminate fruit as a food choice and that is not something you want to do. What you *do* want to do is cut down on the carbs you eat. Try not to eat as much and, when you do, make sure they are from the right sources.

Carbs in white bread, traditional pasta and other processed sources can be harmful, not only because of the carb count but also because of the sugar they have in them. This sugar is often hidden and something people don't even think about. They are used to the sweetness of their sandwich bread, thus they wouldn't think there was any sugar in it. When you are cutting carbs, you may find that you are having sugar cravings.

The easiest way to cut these sugar cravings is to consume sweetness but of the right kind of sweetness source. If you find you are getting sugar cravings very often, you should eat a piece of fruit. The fruit will allow you to get the sugar you need and help cut the cravings. Fruit will keep you from bingeing on unhealthy food and help you feel better about what you are eating.

Water

Since your body is made up of mostly water, it would make sense that consuming water is going to keep you healthy. Water is the *only* thing humans should be drinking. The body was designed to consume water. It wasn't designed to consume soda, fruit juices, tea or even coffee. While these can be hard habits to quit, you should try to rid all of these harmful processed beverages as soon as (or even before) you start to diet. They can be some of the hardest things to quit, but they will allow you to see the biggest change in your belly fat. Even if you are used to drinking diet soda (which is one of the worst processed foods that you can consume), you should stop. Switch all of your drinks to plain water or alkaline water.

While it can be hard at first, water is still the best option. If you are struggling with needing something flavorful, you can make tea or just add lemon slice into your water. You may also make fruit infused drinks. The tea you make should be as blend as possible. To add extra flavor to your tea (or even your water), you can squeeze the juice from one fresh, organic lemon into the drink. It will add extra flavor and help you feel like you are not being deprived of flavorful drinks. The more water you drink, the more you will be able to pick up on different and new flavors in your food. Drinking water before and after meals is one of the best ways to make sure you are able to taste all of the flavors in the food.

Chapter 4: Breakfast Recipes

As the most important meal of the day, you want to make sure you are loading up on all the nutrients that will allow you to make the right choices for the rest of the day. It is a good idea to try out different recipes, but make sure you are eating the things you need to truly lose belly fat. If you add processed foods into it, you will not see the similar positive results, as if you had followed the diet in the right way.

Belly Busting Omelet

Serving Size: 1
Preparation Time: 15 minutes
Ingredients:

2 whites from eggs

1 large white or brown egg

1 tbsp. fresh basil, chopped

1 tsp. lemon zest, grated

1 tsp. lemon juice from a fresh, organic lemon

2 tbsp. Neufchatel cheese

1 tsp. of olive oil

2 oz. spinach, whole leaves

½ cup cooked chicken breast, chopped

Directions: Using a small mixing bowl, put the egg whites, egg, basil, Neufchatel cheese and lemon into the bowl. Add just a tablespoon of water and salt and pepper, if you would like to add some extra flavor. Whisk it until it looks like it is combined and it has been scrambled up. Put a skillet on your stove, over medium heat, with the olive oil in it. Cook your spinach until wilted. Pour the egg mixture into your pan and let it get all over the bottom. Spread the chicken on top of it and fold it over, once the egg has begun to set. Flip it once. Cook for three minutes and serve.

Brunch Quiche

Serving Size: 6
Preparation Time: 30 minutes
Ingredients:

1 tsp. olive oil, darkened

1 broccoli head, cut into smaller pieces

3 whites of eggs

3 brown organic eggs

¾ cup fat-free milk

6 sundried tomatoes, chopped

2 green onions, chopped

¼ cup feta cheese, crumbled

Directions: Heat your oven to 350 F. Use a pie dish to create this recipe and make sure the olive oil has coated both the bottom and the sides of the pan, so you will be able to get the quiche out, without it sticking to the pan.

FCook the broccoli for a few minutes, using either a steamer or in a pan with some water. Do this only until it is soft and not until it is fully cooked. Drain.

Mix eggs, whites and milk together.

Put broccoli and tomatoes into the mixture and stir gently. Add the spring onions and feta and stir once more.

Pour the mixture into the pie dish. Place dish in the preheated oven and bake for about 30 minutes.

If it is not set when you look at it, bake a little longer, perhaps in 5-10 minute increments, until set.

Remove from oven and let rest for 5 minutes. Slice into 6 pieces and serve.

Oats on the Go

This is a protein and fiber rich breakfast that is great for when you are on the go. Use it if you have to eat on your way to work, if you are in a hurry in the morning or if you just want something that is cold and fresh in the morning. You can also change this up and put any type of fruit you want in it. Bananas and natural peanut butter are a great combination for breakfast and will add even more protein.

Serving Size: 1
Preparation Time: 10 minutes
Ingredients:
5 strawberries, chopped into smaller pieces
10 ripe blueberries
2 tbsp. natural rolled oats or steel cut oats (not instant)
½ cup Greek yogurt (homemade or natural/organic purchased)
1 tsp. natural honey (not the kind that comes in a bear bottle), organic is best

Directions: Put half of each of the berries into the bottom of a lidded glass jar. Put the oats on top of the berries. Add the yogurt on top of the oats. Add the rest of the berries to the top of the yogurt. Put the lid on it and shake to combine. Allow it to sit in the refrigerator for 8-12 hours but not more than 72 hours.

Nutty Fruity Shake

By cutting up the melon and putting it in the freezer, you are eliminating the need to use ice to make your shake cold, which will cut down on the wateriness of the shake. It is a good idea to freeze more than one serving of this, so you can have the shake any time you want to be able to have a quick breakfast.

This is another good on-the-go breakfast recipe and is great for the drive to work because shakes provide hands-free eating options to you. If you have a vitamin mixer, you can even add this to the single bottle and use it to eat on the go, eliminating one of the steps of the process that would normally require you to put it in a cup and add a straw before you head out the door. If you use this type of mixer, just add a lid and go.

Serving Size: 1
Preparation Time: 5 minutes
Ingredients:
¼ honeydew melon or watermelon, cube and freeze the night before
½ avocado, flesh scooped out of the skin
¼ cup cashews, natural or organic
1 dried date, chopped
1 tbsp. water

Directions: Put all of the ingredients into a blender or a smoothie maker and blend until there are no large chunks in it.

Mexican Eggs

Serving Size: 1

Preparation Time: 30 minutes

Ingredients:

½ organic white or yellow onion, diced

1 tsp. olive oil

¼ chili pepper, seeded and diced

3 eggs

½ avocado, peeled and chopped

Tabasco Sauce with no more than 5 ingredients (most should have 2 ingredients)

Directions: Pour the olive oil into a preheated cast iron skillet and sauté the onion until close to translucent. Add the chili pepper. Sauté the onion and chili pepper for about 1-2 minutes. While cooking, beat the 3 eggs and put them in the pan. Scramble them for as long as you like or until they are no longer runny.

You can actually cook them any way that you like using this recipe and can even make them into an omelet.

Remove eggs from the skillet and put them in a bowl. Top with avocado and tabasco sauce, to taste.

Chia Pudding

Serving Size: 2
Preparation Time: 5 minutes
Ingredients:
¼ cup pomegranate juice
2 tbsp. chia seeds
1 cup homemade Greek yogurt
2 tbsp. pistachios, chopped
2 tbsp. pomegranate seeds

Directions: Before you making this recipe, first make sure the chia seeds are inflated, so they will not expand the recipe. You can do this by mixing the seeds with the pomegranate juice, so they will take on the flavor of the pomegranate. You need to then put them in the refrigerator, so they will be able to expand (usually overnight). Once the chia seeds have expanded, you can start to make the recipe.
Put the combined chia seeds and juice (which should be jelly-like) on the bottom of a glass jar. Put the yogurt on top of it and then put the nuts and pomegranate seeds on top of the yogurt. Seal the jar with the lid and keep it in the refrigerator for up to three days.

Eggy Cups

Serving Size: 12

Preparation Time: 40 minutes

Ingredients:

12 eggs

1 green bell pepper, seeded and diced

1 small Roma tomato, diced

¼ onion, finely chopped

¼ cup fresh cheddar cheese

1 tbsp. olive oil (or all natural olive oil spray)

Directions: Preheat oven to 350 F.

Start out by coating a muffin tin with the olive oil (or olive oil spray). You can avoid this step by using a silicone muffin pan.

Crack eggs into a large mixing bowl and blend or whisk eggs well. None of the yolks should be intact and all should be well combined.

Add the vegetables to the mixture and stir well to combine.

Use an ice cream scoop to get all of the vegetables into each cup evenly and put one scoop in each of the wells of the muffin pan. Top with the cheddar cheese. Place the muffin pan into the oven and bakeF for about 20 minutes or until the egg has set and the cheese begins to brown on top.

Remove from oven and serve.

Healthy Muesli

Serving Size: 2
Preparation Time: 30 minutes
Ingredients:
1 cup old-fashioned oats (not instant)
1 cup organic barley
1 ½ cup water
1 apple, cored and grated
1 banana, peeled and mashed
½ cup yogurt
2 tbsp. cashews
1 tbsp. almonds
1 tbsp. organic or natural honey
1 large cup blueberries

Directions: Add the oats, barley and water to a large glass bowl. Cover it and put in the refrigerator for at least 8 hours, but overnight works best. Allow it to sit for as long as you can, to get the most out of the oats and the barley.

Mix in grated apple and mashed banana with rest of your ingredients together, including the honey, blueberries and nuts.

You can substitute these fruits for other kinds, as well as the nuts. Strawberries and hazelnuts go together surprisingly well.

When all ingredients are combined, you can either serve it cold (which is traditional) or serve it hot by baking in preheated oven at 320 F for 15 minutes so you get a hearty and filling hot breakfast.

This can also be divided it into glass jars with lids and placed in the refrigerator for one of the many on-the-go breakfast choices. If you do this, just make sure that you eat it within three days because the oats and the barley can get too soggy to eat if you leave it for longer.

Chapter 5: Lunch Recipes

Whether you are planning to eat lunch at home, serve lunch up for guests or take your lunch to work, you will be able to make some of these recipes work for you. Each of them is focused on the *Losing Your Belly Diet* and will allow you to stick to your plan, no matter what you doing at lunch. The recipes are so good, they don't even taste like they should be included in a diet cookbook, but they are!

Comfort Soup

Serving Size: 4

Preparation Time: 1 hour

Ingredients:

1 tbsp. olive oil

1 white or yellow organic onion, chopped into 1-inch pieces

1 tbsp. garlic, minced

1 carrot, chopped

64 oz. chicken stock

1 cup lentils

½ cup brown rice

1 bay leaf

1 tbsp. fresh thyme leaves, chopped

4 tbsp. juice of a fresh lemon

Directions: In a large stock pot, heat olive oil over medium heat. Add onion and garlic and cook for about 3 minutes, before the onion begins to turn translucent. Add carrot to pot and cook for about 2 minutes. Then, add chicken stock and the rest of the ingredients, except for the lemon juice.

Cook for 40 minutes or until it looks like the rice and lentils are beginning to soften up. Take the bay leaf out of the pot and discard it.

Add the lemon juice and cook for another 5 minutes, to allow it to incorporate. Serve hot.

Southern Europe-Style Salad

Serving Size: 2
Preparation Time: 30 minutes
Ingredients:
½ head romaine lettuce
3 Roma tomatoes, diced
1 cucumber, diced
1 yellow bell pepper, diced
1 orange bell pepper, diced
½ red onion, sliced thin
1 small can of sliced black olives
1 tbsp. olive oil
4 tbsp. fresh basil, chopped
4 tbsp. dried parsley
4 tbsp. balsamic vinegar
Pinch salt and pepper
¼ cup feta cheese, crumbled

Directions: Start out by making the salad. Make sure the lettuce has been rinsed, spun, dried and chopped into smaller pieces, but not as small as the other vegetables. Add the rest of the vegetables, including the olives, to the salad and place it all into two different large bowls. Mix it up and toss it, so all of the vegetables are combined and the flavors are mixed.

In a medium-sized bowl, combine the basil, the parsley, the olive oil, the vinegar and the salt and pepper. Use a whisk to make sure the oil and vinegar are well combined.

Pour the dressing over the salad and mix, using a fork or tongs. Top with feta cheese and serve right away.

If you are not going to serve right away, leave the feta and the dressing off of the salad to help keep it as crisp as possible.

Turkey with Fruit Relish

Serving Size: 2
Preparation Time: 30 minutes
Ingredients:

1 tbsp. olive oil

2 large pieces turkey

1 tsp. seasoned salt

1 grapefruit, peeled and chopped

½ avocado, peeled and chopped

1 green onion, finely chopped

1 tbsp. chopped fresh cilantro

1 tsp. red wine vinegar

1 tsp. honey

Directions: Heat olive oil in a large skillet, over medium heat. Coat turkey with the seasoned salt and place it into the pan. Allow the turkey to get slightly crispy on the outside, so that the flavors are infiltrating the turkey. Once it is slightly crispy on both sides of each slice of turkey (approximately 2 to 3 minutes), remove it from the pan and set it aside on the plates you will be serving on.

Add the rest of the ingredients to a blender and pulse for 10-second increments. You do not want to make a puree, but do want to be sure everything is small and well blended. It should only take about 4 pulses for this to happen.

Pour the relish from the blender into a small pot and stir it, to be sure that everything, especially the honey, is well incorporated. Heat it to a simmer and allow the relish to simmer for about 5 minutes, to further incorporate the flavors and become more jellylike.

When finished, remove from the heat and pour the relish over each of the pieces of turkey, dividing it evenly.

Serve hot or store the relish separately from the turkey, if making a take-along lunch for work. Just add the relish to the turkey before reheating, to make sure the flavors blend together but not too much.

Unique Quinoa

Serving Size: 3
Preparation Time: 30 minutes
Ingredients:

1 ½ cups water

1 cup quinoa (natural or organic), rinsed

1 cucumber, chopped

1 bell pepper (any color), chopped

2 cups cherry tomatoes, chopped

½ cup feta cheese, crumbled

1 tbsp. fresh mint

2 tbsp. apple cider vinegar

Directions: Place the water and quinoa into a large pot and bring it to a boil for about 10 minutes. It should begin to get larger when it is ready to eat.

While the quinoa is cooking, mix all of the vegetables into a large bowl. Combine well and add the feta cheese, making sure it is also well incorporated with the vegetables. Add the rest of the ingredients and combine well to blend flavors. The mint and the vinegar should be combined beforehand to make a sauce that you can add to the mixture and put it together.

Once your quinoa has cooked, add it to the vegetable mixture and stir until combined nicely.

Serve hot or cold.

Rollups

Serving Size: 1

Preparation Time: 10 minutes

Ingredients:

3 tbsp. cream cheese, softened

1 tsp. lime juice

1 tbsp. fresh dill, finely chopped

6 slices prepared natural ham

6 very small cucumbers, skin removed

Directions: Start by mixing the cream cheese, lime juice and dill. This will create something of a sauce that you will place on the ham. Lay out the pieces of ham on a baking sheet or a plate and spread the cream cheese mixture onto each of the pieces, so they are covered. On each slice of ham, place one cucumber on top of the cream cheese and roll up the sides of the ham. Secure it with a toothpick. Serve immediately or keep in the refrigerator for up to one day.

Pepper Pine nut Salad

Serving Size: 2
Preparation Time: 30 minutes
Ingredients:
½ head romaine lettuce, washed, dried and chopped
2 bell peppers (two different colors), finely sliced
¼ red onion, finely sliced
1 tbsp. olive oil
1 lemon (organic), juiced
2 tbsp. fresh basil, chopped
2 tsp. pine nuts
Salt and pepper, to taste

Directions: Start off with making the dressing and the garnishes.

To make the dressing: mix the lemon juice with the olive oil. Add salt and pepper to taste, if you want it to pick up some of the other flavors.

In a small pan over medium heat, with a small amount of olive oil, toast the pine nuts until golden.

Place washed, dried and chopped lettuce in medium bowl. Put the onions and the peppers on top of the lettuce.

Pour the prepared dressing over the salad and garnish it with the basil and toasted pine nuts.

If planning to take this to work or you just want it is as crispy as possible, save the dressing and the pine nuts until you are ready to eat, then put them on top so the lettuce and other vegetables do not wilt because of the dressing and nuts.

Dill Salmon

Serving Size: 1

Preparation Time: 30 minutes

Ingredients:

1 salmon filet

1 tbsp. fresh organic lemon juice

1 tsp. fresh dill, finely chopped

1 tbsp. Neufchatel cheese

Directions: Brush the salmon with the lemon juice on both sides of the filet. Preheat your outdoor grill to about 400 F. Spray the grill grate (prior to heating) with a natural olive oil spray or coat it with olive oil.

Once the grill is hot, lay the salmon down on the grill and allow it to cook for about 4 minutes on one side. Flip it and cook on the other side for another 4 minutes. The outside of the filet should be somewhat flaky and cooked the whole way through. Plate it and allow it to rest for a few minutes.

Meanwhile, combine the Neufchatel cheese with the dill to create a spread. Cover the salmon with the spread and serve.

You can serve it with fresh vegetables – peppers and onions work great on their own or even over a bed of couscous.

There are many different options for this lunch dish. Ideally, it should be eaten immediately for the best taste and so you be sure it is the right temperature, and it does not become soggy from the cream cheese mixture. Because it is salmon, make sure that you serve it within a day or two of making it, so that it does not start to go bad.

Chapter 6: Dinner Recipes

Dinner time is usually a time reserved for families to come together and enjoy a meal, as a family, but that can be difficult to do if you are trying to diet. The nice thing about the *Lose Your Belly Diet* is that you don't have to worry about special mixes, shakes or even recipes to eat for dinner. All of the recipes you can eat on the *Lose Your Belly Diet*, you can also serve to your family. The best part is that you will not even feel guilty about serving them delicious food because it is good for them, too!

Chicken Starter

Serving Size: 8

Preparation Time: 30 minutes

Ingredients:

8 oz. cherry tomatoes, cut into halves

4 tbsp. olive oil

2 tbsp. garlic, minced

2 tbsp. tarragon, finely chopped

1 tbsp. chili pepper flakes

4 chicken breasts

Directions: Preheat oven to 400 F.

Mix the tomatoes, olive oil and garlic together. Add half of the tarragon and the chili flakes in with the mixture.

Lay the chicken down in a glass baking dish that has a bit of olive oil rubbed on the bottom to keep it from sticking.

Pour the tomato and garlic mixture over top of the chicken and make sure it is covered completely. Place in preheated oven and roast for 30 minutes.

When cooked through, the chicken should have juices that are running clear. Make sure the chicken is still covered with the cooking juice and tomatoes.

Top with the remaining tarragon and serve.

You can then use leftover chicken for other recipes or serve it with vegetables and brown rice to round out the meal.

Protein Bake

Serving Size: 4
Preparation Time: 1 hour
Ingredients:
1 cup cooked red kidney beans (canned are OK, but dried and cooked are better)
2 cups dried lentils
3 cups water
1 tbsp. olive oil
1 onion, chopped
1 tbsp. garlic, minced
2 Roma tomatoes, diced
2 handfuls shredded kale
2 tsp. Creole seasoning
1 tsp. salt
1½ cupnatural aged sharp cheddar cheese, grated

Directions: Preheat oven to 400 F.
After making sure kidney beans are cooked, begin cooking the lentils. In a large saucepan, bring water to a boil, add lentils and boil for about 15 minutes. This will ensure that the lentils are as soft as possible. Drain the lentils and put them to the side with the cooked beans.
Pour olive oil into a preheated iron skillet, add onion and garlic and sauté for about 5 minutes, or until translucent. Do not allow to burn.
Add the tomatoes and kale. Sprinkle the Creole seasoning and salt onto the vegetables and allow to cook for 10 minutes, over medium

heat.

Add lentils and kidney beans to the mixture and stir together. Sprinkle cheese on top.

Place the cast iron skillet into the preheated ovenF and bake for 20 minutes or until the cheese is completely brown. If you want a crispy top, use the broiler for about 2 minutes to make sure the cheese gets crispy.

Steak Bites and Couscous

Serving Size: 4
Preparation Time: 30 minutes
Ingredients:

1 top sirloin steak

⅓ cup olive oil

½ cup soy sauce

¼ cup Worcestershire sauce

1 tbsp. garlic, chopped

1 tbsp. parsley, dried

1 tbsp. basil, dried

1 cup cooked couscous

1 onion, sliced

1 green pepper, sliced

1 tsp. olive oil

Salt and pepper

Directions: Start out by making the marinade for the steak. Mix the olive oil, soy sauce and Worcestershire together, in a small mixing bowl. Add the garlic, basil and parsley into the mixture. Whisk to combine.

Place the steak and the marinade into a zipper-style plastic bag and allow it to marinate in the refrigerator overnight. If you do not have enough time to marinate overnight, allow it to marinate for no less than three hours.

Preheat the oven to 400 F.

Before you begin cooking the steak, prepare the vegetables. Slice your onions and peppers so they are roughly the same size, place them in a bowl and coat them with the olive oil. Spread them out on a baking sheet in one, even layer. Sprinkle with salt and pepper, to taste, and put them in the preheated oven for about 15 minutes. They should become very fragrant as they cook.

On the stove, heat up a drizzle of olive oil in a cast iron skillet on medium heat. Make sure it is hot before you lay the steak in it. Brown the steak for 1 minute on each side, about 2 minutes total.

Cut the sirloin steak into small pieces.

Take the vegetables out of the oven and lay the steak on top of them. Allow to cook together for about 8 minutes or until it has reached your desired doneness.

Serve the steak and vegetables on top of the previously prepared couscous.

Better than Chicken Noodle

Serving Size: 8
Preparation Time: 1 hour
Ingredients:

1 tsp. of olive oil

½ medium onion, chopped

1 tsp. ground ginger

2 tsp. garlic, chopped

2 small green chilies

½ tsp. ground turmeric

1 tsp. salt

½ tsp. cumin

2 cups dried green lentils

2 cubes organic chicken stock, 20g

2 chicken breasts, cooked and diced

1 tbsp. lemon juice

2 tbsp. fresh cilantro, roughly chopped

Directions: Heat olive oil in a small sauce pan, over medium heat. Add the onion and cook about 3 minutes or until beginning to turn translucent - don't let it start to burn. Add the ginger, garlic, and chilies to the pan and stir. Sauté until done the cooking for approximately 1 minute. Finally, stir in the turmeric, salt and cumin.

Place onion and chili mixture into a large stock pot, add the lentils and chicken stock. Cook on high until it starts to boil, about 5 minutes, then reduce the heat and allow to simmer. Add the chicken and continue to simmer for 40 minutes until the chicken gets even softer and the lentils are as soft as possible. Take the soup off the heat and allow it to cool for a few minutes. Add the lemon juice, top it with cilantro leaves and serve.

German Vegetable Mix

Serving Size: 2
Preparation Time: 30 minutes
Ingredients:
1 quart jar of natural sauerkraut, drained and squeezed to get all of the juice out
1 organic white onion, chopped
2 stalks celery, chopped
1 green pepper, chopped
1 small jar diced pimentos, juice drained
1 tsp. yellow mustard
½ cup olive oil
½ cup apple cider vinegar

Directions: Place sauerkraut and the rest of the vegetables into a large glass mixing bowl. This will allow you to combine everything well. Once mixed well, put aside.

On the stove, heat olive oil and vinegar in a small saucepan, over medium heat. Allow the mixture to come to a boil to help thicken it. As soon as it starts to boil, take it off of the heat. Pour mixture on top of the vegetables and combine.

Cover the bowl to store and so as not to ruin the smell of your refrigerator. You can store this salad for up to a week. But make sure you give it at least one hour after you initially make it, before eating it, so that the flavors are all able to come together.

Diet Style Ratatouille

Serving Size: 6

Preparation Time: 1 hour

Ingredients:

1 head cauliflower, cut into florets 3 bell peppers (red, orange and yellow), chopped

½ red onion, thinly sliced

2 medium zucchinis, washed and diced

1 tbsp. olive oil

1 tbsp. thyme, dried

1 tbsp. rosemary, dried

2 tbsp. parsley, dried

Directions: Preheat oven to 400 F.

Bring a pot of water to a boil, place cauliflower in the water to blanch - do not cook it to the point of being soft - but make sure it has been able to sit in the boiling water for a few minutes. Remove it from the water, drain it and allow to dry. You may need to pat it dry twice, to remove any moisture from it, before mixing it with the rest of the vegetables.

Place the dry, blanched cauliflower, along with the other vegetables, in a glass baking dish, making sure they are in a single layer. Do not allow the vegetables to lay on top of each other because they might not fully cook. Drizzle vegetables with olive oil and mix. Sprinkle the thyme, rosemary and parsley on top of the vegetables and put them in the oven.

Roast for about 30 to 40 minutes, or until the cauliflower is soft.

Cauliflower is the hardest of the vegetables, so make sure it is cooked to desired doneness.

Serve with brown rice, couscous or any meat of your choice that is in line with the *Lose Your Belly Diet*.

Chapter 7: Snack and Drink Recipes

If you get hungry between meals, don't reach for the candy bar or drive to the fast food restaurant. The following drinks and snacks are the perfect way to curb your hunger and make sure you are feeling good enough to continue your day without blowing your diet. Use the snacks on their own, in combination with other food you have or even as a side dish with one of the other recipes in this book. Keep in mind with the drinks that everything should be in moderation. Keep your portions small and give yourself a chance to see what the drink is really like, before guzzling it down.

Carrots with Ginger

Serving Size: 4

Preparation Time: 30 minutes

Ingredients:

1 bag carrots, 16 oz., peeled and cut into small strips

2 tbsp. olive oil

2 tbsp. garlic, minced

1 tsp. ground ginger

1 tbsp. poppy seeds

1 tsp. black pepper

Directions: Preheat the oven to 250 F.

In a large mixing bowl, mix all of the ingredients, except for the carrots, until well combined and flavors are blended. Add the carrots to the mixture and do your best to coat them well.

Place all of the carrots, in a single layer, on a large baking sheet, making sure they are not overlapping each other. FPut the carrots into the oven and allow them to cook for about 20 to 30 minutes, or until you have a dried-style carrot. Remove from oven and allow to cool.

When completely dried and cooled, you can then put them into bags and use them to snack on, any time you like.

Healthy Devils

Serving Size: 10

Preparation Time: 30 minutes

Ingredients:

5 eggs, hard boiled and peeled

2 avocados, halved, pitted, flesh scooped out mashed

1 tbsp. garlic, minced

1 tbsp. olive oil

Salt and pepper, to taste

Directions: Start out by hard boiling eggs in a large pot. If the pot is at a rolling boil, it should only take about 10-12 minutes to be sure the eggs are completely cooked through. It is a good idea to then place the eggs in an ice bath, so they are easier to peel. Peel the eggs and cut each of them in half, gently removing the yolks from the whites.

Place the yolks into a large mixing bowl. Rinse the egg whites off, so there is no yellow on them anywhere and arrange them on a large plate, in a circle.

Add the avocado, garlic, olive oil and spices to the mixing bowl with the yolks. Blend until well combined, making sure there are no big chunks of egg yolk in the mixture. If the mixture seems a little dry, you can add a little dash of olive oil and blend again. No more than a small amount will be needed. Then, spoon the yolk mixture into the egg whites and serve. They work as both a snack and as a party food.

Smoothie with Mango

Serving Size: 1
Preparation Time: 5 minutes
Ingredients:

½ mango, cubed

½ cup Greek yogurt

1 cup coconut water

¼ tsp. ground cardamom

1 tsp. organic honey

Directions: Make sure that all of your ingredients are prepared and get your blender or your food processor out.

Put all of the ingredients into your blender, making sure they are in the correct order to be able to use the blender the right way.

Blend on chop or by pulsing for around 30 seconds at a time, until thoroughly blended.

Make sure that there are no big chunks of anything in the smoothie before you serve it.

Zucchini Bites

Serving Size: 4

Preparation Time: 30 minutes

Ingredients:

2 small zucchinis, halved lengthwise

1 tsp. olive oil

¼ tsp. seasoning salt

For the salsa:

1 tbsp. cilantro, fresh chopped

1 green onion, finely diced

½ can crushed pineapple (2 oz.), drained

1 tsp. fresh ginger, grated

1 chili pepper, finely diced

1 onion, finely diced

2 tsp. of olive oil

2 tsp. of soy sauce

3 tbsp. fresh organic lime juice

Directions: Preheat the grill to 200 F.

In a small glass mixing bowl or on a plate, coat zucchini with 1 tsp. olive oil and the seasoning salt.

FLay prepared zucchini on the grill, flesh facing up. Cook for about 2 minutes on each side and then remove from the grill. Allow it to sit, until you finish making the salsa to go on top.

In a small bowl, mix all of the salsa ingredients together, until well combined. Serve zucchini with salsa on top.

Summer Smoothie

Serving Size: 1

Preparation Time: 10 minutes

Ingredients:

1 ¼ cup mixed berries (blueberries, strawberries, raspberries, etc.), rinsed and stems removed

¾ cup homemade Greek yogurt

1 orange, juiced and seeds strained out

1 tbsp. organic honey

½ tsp organic vanilla extract

Directions: Put all of the ingredients into a clean blender or a smoothie maker, making sure there are no orange seeds or berry stems. Blend until smooth.

You can also substitute other ingredients like bananas and kiwis or even use lemon juice for something that tastes similar to a frozen lemonade.

If you want to make a shake instead of a smoothie, just freeze your Greek yogurt in ice cube trays, so it is easy to throw into the smoothie.

Put the smoothie into a jar and refrigerate for up to three days. You can take it to work or on-the-go with you.

Small Spinach

Serving Size: 20
Preparation Time: 30 minutes
Ingredients:

1 tbsp. olive oil

1 onion, finely diced

1 tbsp. garlic, minced

1 large chili pepper, finely chopped

1 handful of baby spinach, whole

1 small container of cottage cheese

1 egg

1 tbsp. organic parmesan cheese, grated

½ cup whole wheat bread crumbs

Directions: Preheat oven to 350 F.

Heat the olive oil in a pan, over medium heat. Add the spinach and cook until it begins to wilt. Once wilted, remove from heat and let it cool for a few minutes.

Place cooled spinach in a large mixing bowl, along with the remaining ingredients. Mix until combined well. Form mixture into 20 balls Fand place them on a baking sheet or two.

Place the baking sheet(s) into the oven and bake for about 20 minutes or until the balls start to get crispy.

Move the sheet(s) to the top rack and broil for about 1 minute to add some additional crispiness to the bites. Remove from oven, cool and serve; or store for future use.

Chapter 8: How Should I Feel After Detox?

Once you have made the decision to start the *Lose Your Belly Diet*, you will need to make sure that you detox. Detoxing is a vital part of gut restoration and will help you to be sure that all of the toxins and chemicals from processed foods are out of your system. It will also ensure that you are getting the most out of the diet, as the hardest part will be over before you even start the diet itself. The detox is difficult, but it will be worth it.

Immediately After
The detox part of the diet is one of the hardest parts and the longer you have been eating unhealthily, the more difficult it will be. One word of caution is to <u>not</u> binge on processed foods, before you decide to detox, because it will be harder for your body to get rid of that high load of toxins.

As soon as you come out of the detox phase, you will feel better. This could be because you are comparing it to how terrible you felt while doing the detox, but you will also notice a renewed sense of energy and a desire to continue this healthy eating, so you do not go back to the unhealthy ways and have to do the same type of detox again. The rest of the diet should not be hard for you to manage, compared to the problems that will come with detox.

New Beginnings
This is just the beginning of your new healthy lifestyle, and should

help you see that things are only going to get better, the more you start to eat healthily and work to reduce the belly fat you have previously acquired. The diet is easy to do, once you have completed detox, and keeping track of your new beginnings is a great way to stay on track.

At some point, the diet may become boring or monotonous, especially if you do not try all the different foods available. This is not a problem, except that it could cause you to go back to old eating habits. During this time, you want to make sure you keep in mind the way you felt when you first came out of detox. You felt great - like it was a new beginning! Remember this and allow yourself the chance to improve things with your diet. You will be great and things will be better.

Toilet Habits

One of the first things you will notice with the detox process is that your toilet habits will immediately change. Toilet visits can get more frequent and it is a perfectly normal way for your body to rid the toxins and waste accumulated overtime.

Reduced Stress and Anxiety

It is easy to see that your life will be significantly better when you come out of detox, and you can make more decisions about the healthy lifestyle you have chosen. One thing that may surprise you is that you will have a reduced amount of stress. The diet is aimed at making sure you reduce stress, because cortisol is bad for your body. Losing weight, learning clean eating habits and doing more with your body will all contribute to better health and a better attitude about the life you are living.

Reduced stress will also lead to less anxiety and other mental health problems. There are many people who have a lot of anxiety and do not know why. It most often comes from the way they eat. Changing your eating habits will reduce your stress, which will, in turn, help to reduce the anxiety you have on a daily basis, and give you a renewed sense of gratefulness for the life you have.

While changing the way you eat may not be able to cure you of any mental illnesses you have, it can't hurt them either. You will see that things can get better with any mental illness, when you have a healthy diet. Even if you are currently medicated for your mental illness, changing your eating habits will help you learn that you can manage many different things when it comes to your mental health.

A More Focused Attitude

Losing weight, alone, is enough to help you have a better attitude and be more focused on the different things you can do. There are many things you will be able to focus on, and it will give you the chance to make sure that you are doing everything the right way. When you are eating healthy, you can focus on important goals, deadlines and dreams you may have. You will be able to see that there is a lot that comes from healthy eating and your mind will be sharper too.

The toxins in the processed foods are literally poisoning your brain, which is causing you to have slower response times, a harder time concentrating and a more difficult outlook on life. It can be a problem for many people who want to make sure they are doing things the right way. You will be more efficient at everything in life, when you cut out the processed foods and the toxins that come along with them. You will have the chance to do the most with what you have to offer. You will be able to learn as much as possible about the world around you, when you are able to truly focus on it, instead of focusing on how terrible you feel from processed foods.

Less Hunger

It may seem counterintuitive to be less hungry when you are dieting, but the *Lose Your Belly Diet* isn't just another fad. It is a change in your lifestyle and is something in which you will actually see the difference, when you are doing the diet. You will be less hungry and fuller all the time, instead of always wanting to eat something because of the way processed food leaves you.

The *Lose Your Belly Diet* puts a lot of focus on the protein and fiber available in different foods. These are both important options and will allow you to stay fuller longer. Protein and fiber will not leaving you feeling stuffed, in the way that processed carbs do, but will assure that you are truly full. The more protein and fiber you consume, the longer you will be able to stay satisfied and keep hunger at bay. There are many benefits to consuming more fiber and protein but this is one of the best ones. This diet will allow you to feel satisfied and seldom hungry.

Improved Taste

The same toxins that dull your mind in the processed foods are the ones that will also have negative effects on your taste buds. They become numb to the point that you really can't taste the flavor of different things. They are altered but easily fixed, once you have detoxed out of the processed food lifestyle. You will need to make sure that you are getting the most out of your new healthy food lifestyle, by always trying new things and new flavors that contribute to your taste buds being renewed.

There are many different flavors you could be missing out on because your taste buds are numb, due to the toxins in fast foods and processed foods. Make sure you try new things, after you have fully detoxed. You may be surprised to find food tastes much better or it has a different taste from the way you imagined in the past. Even water will take on a new taste and will leave you feeling like it is something delicious, instead of un-flavorful.

Lighter

The most obvious thing that will happen when you detox is that you will be physically lighter. You will lose weight from the detox alone and that should prepare you to lose even more when it comes time to start the actual *Lose Your Belly Diet*. Losing weight through the detox will be the largest amount of weight you lose, at one time, during the diet. It is rapid and will leave you much lighter than when you were eating processed foods. It will also give you the chance to get what you need nutrient wise.

Not only will you be physically lighter but you will also *feel* lighter. The processed food can weigh you down, make you feel heavy and make you feel sluggish. When you switch away from processed foods, during the detox, you will begin to feel lighter. Even though you may feel much worse for a few days, while you are detoxing, it is important to note that this is only a part of the process and it will get better. You will feel bad because the toxins are leaving your body, but once they have left and your detox is finished, you will feel lighter.

More Eager to Begin

Once you have completed the detox, you will see all of the benefits that come along with it. This will allow you to see that the diet will be great and you will truly get a lot of different benefits from the diet as well. You may be prepared for the diet when you start the detox, but after the detox, you will be eager to begin.

This eagerness does not just come from the fact that you will be able to place delicious foods back into your diet, but it also comes from the fact that things can be so much better after the detox.

Make sure you are prepared for the diet by doing the detox. While it may seem intimidating at first, the detox is worth it, if you want to make sure you are getting the most out of the *Lose Your Belly Diet* and are living your healthiest life.

Chapter 9: Sustaining Your Belly Free Lifestyle

After you have done the detox, you may think it is free sailing from there. You aren't wrong, as long as you are able to follow the *Lose Your Belly Diet* guidelines. Make sure you only eat food that is approved and will be nourishing to you. Don't fall off of the wagon and go back to the processed foods while you are dieting. Always make sure you are trying your best to cook everything on your own. The diet is focused around healthy and natural choices, so always try to incorporate those ideas into your diet. This will ensure that you are eating the right way and are able to get the most out of what you have accomplished.

Once you have completed the diet, it may be easy to fall back into your old ways. While you are maintaining your weight, it is acceptable to eat a processed food every once in a while, but you should not go back to the way you were. You need to constantly work at maintaining your new lifestyle and focus on each of these points when you are trying to sustain it, without the big belly following you...or leading you around.

Watch Your Portions
Once you have completed the initial diet phase of dieting, it can be easy to get carried away with the food you are going to eat. You should make sure that you keep your portion sizes about the same as when you were losing weight and getting rid of your belly. The nice thing about the *Lose Your Belly Diet* is that you are able to eat

healthy food until you are satisfied, instead of just eating a little bit of food here and there. Keep in mind the satisfaction you get from food and what it feels like. This is important when you are maintaining your weight, so you will be able to know when to stop.

Even though your portions can be slightly larger than when you were losing weight, they shouldn't be too much larger. This is something you need to always work at and try to avoid. If you are allowing your portions to get too big, you may be overeating.

The point of the diet is to teach you to avoid overeating, not continue doing it when you are trying different things. It is important that you make the choice to always try different things and that you don't eat too much. It can be detrimental to your body and to your waistline to do this. Too much food at one time can weigh you down and make you too full. Even if you are eating healthy food, huge portions can wreak havoc on your gut, and you will need to start over from the beginning with the gut health work you did when you first began the diet.

The Work Isn't Done
You will always need to pay close attention to your weight and the size of your belly. Don't let it get out of hand, no matter how far you are into sustaining a healthy lifestyle. Constantly work at getting healthier and making the right choices. Consider the exercise options you have when you are trying to maintain your weight. This will enable you to get the most out of the work you've done. You should be careful with what you are doing when it comes to food.

One thing you may want to do is always check your gut health. Be aware of what gut health should mean to you and what can happen if you get too much bad bacteria in your gut. This can be a problem and it can cause you a lot of pain and hassle. Watch your bathroom habits and make sure they are staying the same as when you were dieting.

If you find that you do not have a very happy or healthy gut, you will need to take the time and retry the four R's. This will help you to restore your gut. It can be hard to do this after you have already started to maintain your healthy lifestyle, but it will be worth it for you.

Before you get to this point, be sure you are still consuming plenty of Greek yogurt and other sources of good bacteria. If you started with a clean slate of no bacteria in your gut, the good bacteria should be able to overpower the bad and make sure they are not present or harming you.

Cook at Home
With the hustle and bustle of everyday life, it can be easy to get caught in the trap of eating out. Even when you eat at a healthy restaurant or you choose to make healthy choices at an average restaurant, things can become unhealthy really quickly. The main goal of trying to make sure you are doing the right thing is to try to eat at home or at least cook at home, most of the time. This will ensure that you are doing things the right way and that you know where your food is coming from.

When you cook your food at home, you know exactly what is in it.

This is especially true if you are preparing it all yourself and not using packaged food. This is even truer if you are making things on your own, like Greek yogurt. Knowing where the food comes from and that there are no added ingredients or trans fats in the food, can be the difference in maintaining a healthy life and seeing all the weight that you dropped so fast come right back in the way it did in the beginning.

If you find that you are struggling with eating out, consider some of the other options you have. There are many snacks you can choose from that you can keep in your car or close to you while you are at work. They can work much better than eating out. Another option is to prepare all of your lunch meals and even some of your dinner meals ahead of time, so you do not have to worry about trying to find something to eat last minute and then eating out because there was nothing prepared at home.

Avoid Fast Food

It doesn't matter if you have been maintaining your weight for 10 days or 10 years, fast food is always going to be a bad idea. Not only is fast food poison but it is also addictive. The first time that you dive into a big box of greasy fries after you have dieted for so long, you will be miserable within a few hours. The problem is that you will want more. The hydrogen that is in the trans fat and all of the other mystery additives can cause you to get addicted to the fast food in the same way that your brain can get addicted to other things.

Any type of restaurant is better than the fast food kind. While fast food restaurants are the worst, chain restaurants are almost just as bad because of the additives they put into their food and the way in which the food is made. It is also important to note that you can choose a family-owned restaurant or something similar, over a chain restaurant, and it will be much healthier for you. Family-owned restaurants will be the healthiest option of all of them, unless there is a natural, organic or health-based restaurant that you can go to. If this is an option, always choose it.

If you have absolutely no choice but to eat at a fast food restaurant, try to find something that is not cooked. Try a salad or a fruit packet, if it's an option. These likely still have the preservatives in them but they probably do not have as many additives as, say, a burger would have. Another option, at some fast food restaurants, is to try a baked potato instead of fries.

Don't Overdo the Drinks

When you are dieting, you are limited on what you can drink, when it comes to both alcoholic and nonalcoholic beverages. When it is time to start maintaining the weight you have lost, you may want to make sure you drink as little as possible, other than water, while still being able to enjoy all of the things that come with maintenance. There are many options for you when it comes to this but you should make sure you are getting the most out of it with the diet plan you have.

It may be hard for you to remember that you once could only drink water, so take it easy on the beer, wine and cocktails. While beer and red wine will not be terrible, in moderation, the cocktails could be filled with sugar in addition to the sugar that is in alcohol. If you have not eaten any sugar for a long time, it will be detrimental to your body to try to drink a sugary drink, so be aware of the possible consequences.

One of the worst things that happens while people are trying to maintain their weight is they go back to drinking soda. They think they are in the clear and they can just start drinking soda again. Whether you are drinking diet or regular soda doesn't matter because they are both bad for you. You can start drinking tea, coffee, and even some fruit juices, in moderation, but do your best to stay away from soda. If your only choice is a soda, choose one that is clear and always choose the lowest sugar-filled option of regular over the chemical-filled option of diet.

Try New Things
While you were dieting, you probably tried a lot of new things that you did not think you would enjoy or you had never tried before. This is something that is a major part of dieting and something that will enable you to make better choices for your life. Just because you are in maintenance, does not mean you should stop trying new things. There are probably many things you have never tried; always do your best to branch out.

New recipes are a great way to get yourself to try new things. These can be anything from something that a friend sent you to something you saw on the Internet. But, keep in mind that recipes are not all created equal. Even if you find a recipe that is not quite completely in line with the way you have been eating, you can tweak it to make it friendlier to the *Lose Your Belly Diet,* so you will be able to get the most out of what the diet has to offer.

There are even new foods you can try, without worrying about the new recipes. Chances are that you have not tried *every* fruit or vegetable in the world, so when the opportunity arises, take it and run with it. Trying a new food can be enlightening. Even if it is something you do not think you will like, it won't hurt you to try it. You may even end up with a new favorite healthy food option that you can snack on anytime you like.

Watch Out for Packaged

Similar to how you can get caught up with the eating out problem, it can also be easy to get caught up in buying packaged food again. Be careful that you are not buying packaged food more than you are buying real food. It may be harder for you to have to prepare the food but you will need to make sure you are ready for it before you begin the diet. It may be harder for you, but it will be worth it.

It is not necessarily a bad thing to have a packaged food, once in a while, and it is inevitable that you will need to eat something packaged. One thing you should look out for, always, no matter how often you eat packaged food, is trans fat. Out of all of the additives, carcinogens and the problems that come along with packaged food, trans fat is the worst and it will be the most detrimental to your health and all of the progress that you have made with the *Lose Your Belly Diet*.

Conclusion

Thank for making it through to the end of this book, let's hope it was informative and able to provide you with all the tools you need to achieve your goals, whatever they may be.

The next step is to start figuring out how you are going to do the diet. Check with your doctor before you make the decision to start any diet, but let him or her know that you are planning on making a lifestyle change, instead of doing a fad diet.

Finally, if you found this book useful in any way, a review on Amazon is always appreciated!

www.ingramcontent.com/pod-product-compliance
Lightning Source LLC
Chambersburg PA
CBHW072012290526
45787CB00013B/869